Health Through Fruit

Plant Based Weight Loss and Disease Reversal
Eliminate Eczema, Sinusitis, Lyme Disease,
Autoimmune Diseases, Healthy Birth, Low Fat
High Raw

AMY LYNN HAGER

ISBN: 9881696049436

DEDICATION

I dedicate this book to my family & friends. Thank you for loving
me on my healing journey. You all have truly inspired and
encouraged me to be a better person. Through your love, I have
evolved. I have replaced my fear with love, may you all learn to do
the same! Many blessings on your journey to health. You all deserve
beautiful, healthy lives. I hope this book helps you along your
journey!

CONTENTS

ACKNOWLEDGMENTS

Thank you to Robert Sniadach, Nic La-Paz, Serena La-Paz, Gina Keefe and Darrel Hager for inspiring me, mentoring me and listening to me. You all were either my inspiration or my rock. Thank you for loving me. My journey to health was a painful one but so liberating. I had to let my old self die and be re-born into a new life and.a new way of existing. From the bottom of my heart, thank you! I love my new path. Nothing is better than true health!

I also want to thank you and congratulate you for downloading the book, Health Through Fruit: Plant Based Weight Loss and Disease Reversal (Eliminate Eczema, Sinusitis, Lyme Disease, Autoimmune Diseases, Healthy Birth, Low Fat High Raw)

This book contains proven steps and strategies on how to find health through fruits. You will find your ideal blueprint body weight and learn how to reverse your autoimmune diseases. I've experimented with all sorts of diets and the fruit based diet is the best because of its simplicity, it tastes delicious and fruit is loaded with vitamins and minerals. This is my sweet and tasty plant based path to health and self love. I've poured my heart and soul into this very intimate story about my personal discovery of thriving health. My health journey began when I traveled deep into the magical mountains of Vilcabamba Ecuador after registering for a juicer for my wedding. We sold everything we owned and began our journey of health. Without your health, you have nothing. I hope you enjoy this treasure as much as I did writing it. I dedicate this book to all my beautiful readers whom I love and adore so much. May your health soar as did mine. May you heal yourself with delicious fruits. May you empower yourself to eliminate autoimmune diseases. Many blessing!

Thanks again for downloading this book, I hope you enjoy it! Much love, light and sweet fruit for you all!

INTRODUCTION - DISCOVERY OF SELF HEALING

Hello beautiful people. I have a serious passion for healing of all kinds, mind, body & spirit. This book focuses mostly on the body and a little on the spiritual so that you can make better choices for the body. I see people working out hard for 2 plus hours a day and still not get the results that they desire. I know because I used to be one of those people. I would spend hours at the gym exercising full out and rarely was I happy with my weight and more importantly my health. I needed to clean up my diet. Diet is 70% of your weight issues while working out and daily activities make up the rest. I accidentally stumbled across healthy living by registering for a juicer for my wedding registry at 35. When I got my first juicer I had a blast and looked up tons of videos for recipes. Someone mentioned to me that they met a guy who was on an all raw food diet and how he looked amazing at 60. I could never do that I thought but it sparked my curiosity. I bought a raw food book at a bookstore and was impressed by the bodies ability to heal itself through lifestyle and nutrition. Also, you will find your natural blueprint body weight. That's what I wanted!

I watched my mother suffer from Colitis and Crohn's disease since I was 17 years old. My mother is highly educated with a phD and had a wonderful teaching job with full benefits. I watched her spend millions of dollars on healthcare but she was always in pain, getting a surgery and taking a pill for her aches and pains. I couldn't help but to think, if this was the best that money could buy then it wasn't good enough. There had to be a better way, and there is! I only wish that I had more influence over both of my parents to change their diets and lifestyle. My father has Alzheimer's and his health rapidly declined at 69. There are lots of people out there who want to learn about natural healing and my goal is to reach the ones searching for better health and truth. I would have done anything to help my parents.

I suffered from chronic sinusitis and eczema my whole life and when I read that I could eliminate this through diet I didn't believe it but I had to try it to be sure. How do you know unless you try, right? That is what I was thinking. Six months into my marriage I got pregnant. I had no health insurance and had a sinus infection that lasted a couple months. I couldn't sleep. Both of my nostrils were completely blocked preventing me from breathing out of my nose. I had to sleep with my mouth open which is the worst especially in the morning because I had the driest cotton mouth. This was a chronic condition for me as I would get a sinus infection and traditionally I would take some over the counter pill or antibiotics to get rid of it.

I had a dear friend who had complications with delivering twins. One baby died and one baby lived. I had a lot of fear to prevent any accidents from happening because of her experience. I wasn't going to take any drugs out of fear that it could harm the baby. Not having health insurance ended up being the best thing because I had to learn how to take better care of myself and my family. I found the power of a high raw plant based fruity diet right as I needed to grow a healthy child. I couldn't afford for anything to go wrong. There seemed to be synchronicity in my life where answers were being given right as I needed them.

When I was 7 weeks pregnant I did a 10 day Hypocrites raw food detox to reset my body. I found benefits to this diet while at a health center but I wasn't able to follow through outside of the health center. Hypocrites promotes enemas, wheat grass, fermented foods, sprouts and raw food. One reason why I struggled was that I didn't have access to wheat grass on a daily basis without growing it and juicing it myself. My life is super busy and I need things to be simple. I don't like fermented foods and I don't like sprouts that much. I'm not against enemas but they seem a little unnatural to me. I like microgreens but I really despised the taste of a sprouted lentil or garbanzo bean. I took raw food meal prep courses and a raw food pizza can take 3 days to make!!! Say what?!!! I have to make a crust and dehydrate it for 24 hours and then what?   I am not that organized to prepare all my meals this way nor is it realistic to maintain. I found myself eating a lot of nuts thinking that because it was raw, it was healthy.   Nuts are healthy but in small quantities because of their high fat content and they leave an acidic ash.

I discovered a low fat fruit based diet which I absolutely love. The diet is raw fruits, vegetables, nuts & seeds. I would still eat cooked whole plant based foods occasionally too. I perform the best when I am on this diet athletically and my health soared. I went to fruit lucks and festivals where I met older people who where on a high raw fruit based diet and these guys were amazing! I saw a 74 year old man walk on his hands across the beach. I couldn't even do that! I was seeing people thrive in their older years and I was inspired.

As I was on my health journey, I saw how eating a plant based diet was also good for the planet and the animals. We all can make an impact on changing the world just by changing our diets! Somehow eating this way has guided me toward a path of enlightenment. My spiritual practice has never been stronger and I definitely believe that a healthy vessel brought me closer on my path. As I healed my emotional body then I found it easier to eliminate my addictions, fears and depression, developing clarity. I wish each and everyone of you happy healthy lives and to share this blessing with others. You are a vessel of light. As you are inspired, lead by example and teach someone else how to do it.   I am delighted to share my healing journey with you. Much love and light! Peace.

1 AN INVITATION TO HEALTH - HOW A JOURNEY TO ECUADOR CHANGED MY LIFE

When my ex-husband got sick with Lyme disease, I was 35. He got sick around the time of our wedding. His weight dropped down to 150 lbs at 6'3". We were successfully running a dog training business in Chicago and six months after the wedding I was pregnant. My ex-husband had severe arthritis in his joints that seemed to move around his body without an injury. He also was extremely lethargic and often slept in his car between appointments. He would even be parked in the driveway, sleeping on the wheel because he was too tired to walk inside. It was clear that he needed a break from training dogs because his health was failing him. It was at the height of his business that we worked so hard to grow that we decided to sell. He is an extremely talented dog trainer but his body was inflamed in pain. I thought it was possible that if we didn't make serious changes that he would die. The month that we sold the business we were making $30,000 a month and it was on the verge of doubling. We sold everything that we owned and moved to Vilcabamba Ecuador with a 9 month old baby, 2 dogs and nothing but a suitcase. Vilcabamba is known as the city of longevity, the city of centurions and the fertile valley. It has a comfortable moderate 70 degree year round climate. I knew there was a strong vegan and vegetarian expat community there, as I was watching many of them on youtube. I watched hours of youtube videos on Vilcabamba. I saw there were families living there, working on permaculture farms, plus it was cheap. I knew we had to go to this magical healing place in the middle of nowhere deep in the Andes Mountains.

My ex-husband needed time off to rest and take care of his health. When we were there we found a small Ecuadorian house that was about 2 or 3 blocks away from our new friends Nic from Germany and Serena from Italy. These are two of the most beautiful souls that I ever met. I was on the raw food track but I didn't know much about Natural Hygiene. They were there taking a course from a man named Robert Sniadach at the Transformation Institute. We became friends and they learned that my ex-husband was very sick. They proceeded to tell me about Natural Hygiene and how following this lifestyle would help him boost his immune system and recover his health. They told me that if they ever got really sick that they would immediately do a water only fast followed up by a raw food diet which consists of raw fruits, vegetables, nuts & seeds. The bulk of the calories coming from fruits. We were already vegetarian at this point because of my wedding juicer but we were still eating eggs and dairy. When we heard how a high fruit low fat raw based diet could improve his health, we tried it. He already tried antibiotics but still suffered. The key is to stick with raw fruits and vegetables over time. I learned to eat large quantities of fruits, enough to make a meal and satiate me. Reversing and cleansing the body is not a quick fix. Fasting can help speed up the healing.

I ended up becoming friends with Robert Sniadach and took his Natural Hygiene course. When I started reading it, I was shocked at how detailed and involved the 2000 page course would be. I felt like a doctor reading about the body, the systems, how things worked and how to make the body thrive. As far as I was concerned, Natural Hygiene was the greatest thing that I ever learned. It follows nature and as far as I'm concerned, mother nature didn't mess things up. If we use the simple guideline to follow nature and go back to our roots as a species, then all of us can have thriving health. My ex-husband ended up making a full recovery after 2 years of being debilitatingly sick. My eczema and sinus issues disappeared. Our health improved as we took much needed time off to heal our bodies. My life was forever changed after our move to Vilcabamba. You can't unlearn something. Once you learn about it, there is a truth to it because it follows the laws of nature and the results speak. Following nature makes logical sense. When you try this lifestyle for a period of time, you will feel your health flourish as did mine.

The hardest part about making the lifestyle switch was trying to fit in socially. The world is not healthy. You may lose some friends but you will gain new ones that are aligned with your goals. Unfortunately it is more socially acceptable to go out and get a double bacon cheese burger with fries and a beer or a coke than it is to eat a five mangos or a salad. I was excited to teach everyone back home all about it because I saw many people suffering with illnesses or trauma's and I wanted to help. Most importantly I wanted to heal my mother's Crohn's disease, edema, kidney stones and Parkinson's and my father's Alzheimer's. Other family members suffered too with diabetes, multiple sclerosis, depression, heart issues, obesity and addictions. I was saddened that so many people, including my own parents, didn't want to hear about this healthy lifestyle especially as I watched their health rapidly decline.

I didn't realize what a landmine talking about food was. Lots of people have serious emotional addictions to food. They emotionally medicate themselves through the pleasure of foods that taste good but are not good for them. My friends and family didn't care about healthy living so I had to create my own path alone. I could barely talk about the extensive topic without triggering someone. From my experience people weren't interested in doing their own research on their healthcare. They would only take advice from a doctor which can be a mistake because so many of them are not trained on the health benefits of a plant based diet. The doctors that do recommend this diet are often ignored. People don't want to make changes in their lives because the majority are so brainwashed from a child through television, the school system and society. It's easier to pop a pill or get a surgery but the results are often less than ideal. Let's face it, it's called the healthcare business! People are making a lot of money off of your health. Take back your life, literally. Live free from worry about getting sick. Find the joy in moving your body. Learn how to take care of this magnificent machine that you have been blessed to be given. Don't be another victim to the food industry, the pharmaceutical industry, the medical system, and everyone else looking to make money off of you. Yes, companies will lie to make a profit so learn to see through the lies. What is their agenda? They care about money, not your health. I advise people to really invest in your relationship with your doctor to make sure you find one that knows something about the health benefits of a plant based diet and new research or at least be open minded to learn from you. There are good doctors out there but you have to choose wisely.

For me, if I see an unhealthy doctor, then I am skeptical of their advice. If they can't take good care of their own health then how can they possibly advise me on mine. I say this with caution because we need doctors for medical testing, check-ups and emergencies. The combination of a well-informed doctor and the knowledge of a plant based diet can be a powerful force in the world of healthcare and medicine. It's just sad that the biggest benefactors to medical schools are big pharmaceutical companies, big food corporations, big charities who are in bed with lobbyist. Some of the lobbyist are big time meat corporations, dairy industries and big time anyone who can make a profit by manipulating the government to modify the food pyramid just a little so they can sell more of their products. These lobbyist impact the quality of the education that is taught in medical schools. The topic that is the biggest taboo to talk about and is hardly even taught in medical schools is nutrition. It takes a special doctor who discovers the truth about health and nutrition to be willing to stick their necks out against the grain of social conditioning to offer people truth and real quality healthcare. The sad part about it is that there is more money to be made in what I call the Disease Care System instead of the Health Care System. If you can stay chronically ill but not die, everyone makes money at your expense. It's frustrating to see people I love suffer. I can't help but to think that much of the suffering could have been prevented if there wasn't such a gigantic cluster of contradicting nutritional information forcing people to have to sift through the information to find the truth. I want to give you the truth! It is your birthright to know how to take excellent care of yourself!

2 DISEASE FREE HEALTH IS NORMAL & NATURAL - IT IS YOUR BIRTHRIGHT

We all have a birthright to live a disease free life. It is normal and natural for us to be healthy. Disease is abnormal, unnatural and unnecessary. Disease will not occur unless there is sufficient cause. Why are so many people unhealthy? What is the cause? I work on people regularly doing Thai Yoga Bodywork and I rarely get a pain free healthy person on my mat. So many people are suffering. You won't find many people promoting fruits and vegetables because there is no money in that. It's hard to find the apple lobbyist or the romaine lettuce lobbyist who can cough up as much cash as big corporations for government leaders. In general, I think people are well intentioned but our system is flawed. It's hard to get into office without lobbyist support but at what cost. Greed. We live in a greedy society willing to bulldoze anyone who gets in the way of making profits.

Government subsidies make inorganic and low quality food so cheap. It's hard to get out of a system when the government is supporting industries that cause your illness. Why don't organic farms get subsidies? This makes the healthier food cost more which makes it harder for everyone to buy higher quality foods. We have to make conscious choices to make our health a top priority. We live in our bodies.

There is a significant amounts of brainwashing that happens to all of us from the moment we are born and all through our lives. In public schools, the food they give our children is chosen from the government and it includes an incredible amount of animal products, unripe fruit, not enough fruit and processed foods.   Our food pyramid has been tampered with to accommodate lobbyist in our nutrition classes.   Commercials and tv programs flat out lie to us, "Milk, it does a body good" for example.   No it doesn't.   That commercial needs to say, "Milk, it causes mucus and inflammation". The list of misinformation to overwhelm and confuse the general population regarding nutrition is one of the biggest crimes of all times.   It is up you to wisen up.   Your vote at the grocery store matters. Invest in learning how to take excellent care of yourself and know that you will have to filter through a lot of misinformation to find truth.   There isn't enough money to be made in the truth but your life depends on it.

3 HUMANS AND FRUIT

Fruits are loaded with alkaline minerals which is healing on the body, even citrus. Because citrus has alkaline minerals then even though there is citrus acid in the fruit, it has an alkaline effect on the body. If we look to nature to determine our proper diet then we can see that we are frugivores. There is a law of similars where every animal in the same category eats the same way. For example, all cats eat the same, all horses eat the same, etc. We fall under anthropoid apes and anthropoid apes are fruitarians. We have the same physiology and anatomy. We share the same alkaline digestive systems. We are attracted to their color and sweet taste along with having opposable thumbs which we use to pick and peel it.

Fruit is one of the few foods that we like to eat raw, unprocessed and in its natural form. It is the number one source of vitamins and number two source of minerals for humans. If we were left in a room with grasses, tubers, grains, seeds, animals, vegetables and fruit and had to choose what to eat if we had only our bare hands and no cooking tools then we would choose fruit first and vegetables second. Fruit includes our non-sweet fruits such as tomatoes, zucchini, cucumbers, peppers, okra, etc. There are so many delicious fruits such as apples, oranges, grapes, watermelon, strawberries, mangos, papayas, etc. There is an abundance of tropical fruits that I invite you to seek out and try at some point in your life if you haven't already done so such as jackfruit, durian, longans, lychees, rambutans, sapote, passion fruit, sour sop, sugar apple, mamey, egg fruit, snake fruit, etc. The list is extensive and very delicious. The fragrance of all these fruits is pleasing to our sense of smell. Our digestive physiology is designed to process the soft water-soluble fibers in fruits and tender greens.

Every cell in our human body eats glucose. Fruit has monosaccharides meaning a single simple sugar, readily available for our bodies to use as fuel with minimal processing. Fruit sugars consist of glucose, fructose and galactose. They are pre-digested carbohydrates. Our brain thrives on glucose. If we eat disaccharides (two), polysaccharides (many) or fats then our bodies have to break the chemical structure down into a monosaccharide for our bodies to use as fuel. Monosaccharides can pass through the intestinal barrier and go directly into the bloodstream for use. Disaccharides, polysaccharides, fats and proteins have to be broken down first. 80% of our blood supply is used for digesting foods. When we eat foods that are readily available for our bodies to use with minimal processing then our bodies don't have to work so hard digesting foods. This leaves us with extra energy for healing our bodies and for excelling in our activities and sports. Digestion uses minimal amounts of nerve energy. When we use a lot of nerve energy then that is called "enervating". Enervating means "causing one to feel drained of energy or vitality". A heavy meal that requires a lot of energy to digest is very enervating. Fruits use minimal energy for digestion.

We all consume toxins on a daily basis, from the air, water, foods, etc. When we eat more clean and we use less nerve energy to digest foods therefore our body has extra energy for house cleaning to detox our bodies. There is only one disease, toxicity and a deficiency of vitamins and minerals. Our bodies are always self cleansing and when we conserve energy by eating clean (fruits and vegetables) then we give our bodies this extra energy to heal itself. Nothing heals the body but the body. We cannot out perform mother nature but we can work with her to facilitate our capacity to thrive.

Humans have a sweet tooth for a reason. Fruits satisfy the taste buds on our tongues and are very easy on the digestive system. Enzymes in fruit convert proteins into amino acids and fats into fatty acids and glycerols. All fruits and vegetables contain the three main macro-nutrients carbohydrates, fats and proteins in the correct proportions for humans. Fruits and vegetables are loaded with alkaline minerals such as calcium, potassium, sodium, iron, magnesium and manganese.

Fruit can be eaten as a meal. It is important to eat enough fruit calories to satiate your body. An example is that if you were to eat a diet of 2500 calories then you would need to eat approximately 833 fruit calories for 1 meal if you eat 3 meals a day. If a banana has approximately 80 calories then you would need to eat roughly 10 bananas for breakfast. Not eating enough fruit calories is the biggest mistake that most people make. You can go on sites such as cron-o-meter.com and add up fruit calories, to make sure you are eating enough. Of course like all diets, it is possible to eat too many calories even fruits. Fruits are so low in calories that most of the time this is not the case. If people are not losing weight then most of the time they are eating too much fat in their diet. Bottom line, you need to eat enough calories in for the calories that you use to maintain your weight. When you eat more calories than you use then you gain weight and when you eat less calories than you use then you lose weight. Fruits are 4 calories per gram where fats are 9 calories per gram.

Fruit gets a bad rap due to poor food combining which we will discuss in the next section. Because of food combining rules, the best time of the day to eat fruits are in the morning on an empty stomach. I often eat fruits for lunch as well, especially if I am trying to eat more clean or if I have a busy day because fruits are the easiest and healthiest fast foods available. Any diet that tells you not to eat fruits is a diet that I would stay away from especially since it is one of the best most healing, gentle foods for your body and in nature is one of the few foods that you would eat in its raw natural, unprocessed state.

4 FOOD COMBINING

There is a bio-chemical reaction going on inside your bodies when you eat. The combinations of these foods make digestion more efficient than others. It is not what we eat that determines the nourishment that our bodies receive but rather what we are able to digest and assimilate. Some foods digest faster than others and if they are eaten in poor combinations with food that digests slower then by products such as acetic acids, alcohol and gas are formed. This taxes your kidneys and liver to clean out the blood thus enervating the body. Some foods require a more alkaline stomach to digest such as starches while proteins require a more acidic medium. The stomach has to be very acidic to digest proteins and it neutralizes starch digestion which means undigested food gets moved into the small intestine. Starches like a very alkaline stomach. Starch digestion begins in the mouth where it is mixed with amylase, a starch digesting enzyme. This digestion is arrested if the starch is mixed with a protein that requires the stomach to be acidic. Here are some basic rules:

Eat melons alone and preferably as the first meal of your day. Melons digest the fastest of all your foods because of their high water content.

Eat fruit alone or leave it alone unless combined with celery or lettuce.

Don't combine sweet fruits with acidic fruits. An example is don't combine bananas and oranges together.

Eat starches with vegetables or proteins with vegetables.

Do not mix proteins and starches.

Do not mix sugars with oils.

Sub-acid fruits and acid fruits are a good combination.

Sub-acid fruits and sweet fruits are a fair combination.

Oily foods are avocados, coconuts, olives, nuts and seeds. Oily foods are a good combination with vegetables and starches.

Proteins and oily foods are a poor combination.

The benefits are that you'll have less bloating, indigestion, feelings of dizziness or a simple stomach ache. Because so many people don't know about good food combining then they think it's normal to feel uncomfortable after eating. This is not so, eating is supposed to make you satisfied, filled with good thoughts, emotions and senses. Good food combining can be applied to any any diet to help digest and assimilate foods. Good food combining can help you lose weight, reduce post meal digestive un-ease, improve elimination, resolve skin issues, and to increase energy levels. We all want to feel good right? Well let's recognize the bio-chemical reactions going on in our body and do what we can to help the body digest our foods with ease for our own best comfort.

If you want to eat a meal that is the easiest for your body to digest then consider eating monomeals. A monomeal is eating one food item at a time. An example would be to eat 8 to 12 bananas for breakfast. Or eat 4 or 5 mangos for lunch. Look on cron-o-meter to make sure you are eating enough fruit calories to satiate your body. This is my favorite way of eating and I love the simplicity of it. Going plant based can be scary because you might only think of all the things taken away from you. Consider all the things that are brought into your life. Discover all the fun tropical fruits that there are to enjoy. A fruit meal is fast food. There is no preparation, no

clean up, minimal dishes and it tastes great! I can't emphasize enough
the importance of eating your fruits and in large enough quantities to
make a meal out of them.

5 WHY ACIDIC FOODS ARE HARMFUL?

Our blood wants to maintain a slightly alkaline pH at around 7.4. Coffee is acidic and it's pH is around a 4.5. Some caffeinated soft drinks like Coke is at 2.52 which is very acidic! Your body has five primary alkalizing minerals: Calcium, Magnesium, Potassium, Manganese and Iron. When you drink or eat acidic foods your body dissolves it's alkaline minerals to neutralize the blood pH to maintain homeostasis. Essentially your body is dissolving its bones and minerals into the bloodstream. Your liver and kidney's have to clean the blood which uses nerve energy thus enervating the body. These minerals re-formulate in the kidney's into kidney stones and we pee out our bones. People with Osteoporosis, Anemia or many other diseases would benefit from eliminating all acidic foods while simultaneously eating alkaline foods such as fruits and vegetables. Top acidic foods are meat, dairy, teas, coffees, alcohol, etc. Top alkaline foods are your leafy greens vegetables except spinach, chard, mustard greens and beet greens because they contain oxalic acid in them creating that acidic effect. Stop putting acidic things into the body that your body has to clean up later. Conserve your nerve energy for your sports and activities.

When your body dissolves it's bones to neutralize the blood pH then it can cause arthritis. Let me explain, your body wants to clean the blood all the time. If there are extra minerals in the blood then the body puts them into the places that cause the least damage, your joints. It is also common for calcium deposits to build up in the feet leaving hard bone growths on the feet. This extra calcium build up can come from your water supply as well. Distilled water is best because your body can only absorb organic minerals from plants. Inorganic minerals are plant food, then the plant changes the molecular structure into a format that the human body can easily assimilate. Ideally you are only drinking distilled water when thirsty. When you are eating a lot of fruits and vegetables then you may drink less as there is a lot of hydration in these foods. The more that you cook your foods then the more water you may be drinking since cooking evaporates most of the water from foods. Calcium holds connective tissue in the skin together. When you deplete your skin's calcium then you are causing wrinkles and saggy skin which ages you. If you want to look younger longer, stay away from the acidic foods.

Acidic foods interfere with the digestion of your foods, because they require your stomach to increase the amount of hydrochloric acid in the stomach to digest the foods. This interferes with starch digestion amongst other things. If you eat fruit with acidic foods then it causes the fruit to ferment, releasing acetic acid, alcohol and gas for your liver and kidneys to clean up.

Bottom line, the human digestive system is designed to eat fruits. Fruits are loaded with alkaline minerals which helps replenish the body. We have an alkaline digestive system. Acidic fruits are loaded with alkaline minerals therefore having an alkaline effect on our bodies. So don't be afraid of oranges. They are good for you. They taste good. They smell good so eat them! The more alkaline foods that we eat the healthier that we are going to be. Our blood will be cleaner and we will avoid calcium deposits in the joints, kidneys and skin. Let's face it, good health is attractive. Love yourself enough to give yourself the best. Free up your time working on your health so that you can open your world to all the creative endeavors that are waiting for you on the horizon.

6 TAKE COMMAND OF YOUR HEALTH

I promise you that nobody cares about your health more than you. Nobody knows more about your health than you. If you go to a doctor and a procedure or prescription is recommended then feel free to question things. Do some research and get a second or third opinion. Believe in your ability to take the best care of your body with the advice of qualified individuals and your own research. Remember that natural healing takes time and detox symptoms are not comfortable. They are your body cleansing itself. Detox symptoms can linger and it can be frustrating but hang in there. For me, my health journey has forever changed my life. I feel better than ever and my performance in my sport of choice, yoga, has been excelling even in my 40's. I have been able to successfully reverse my chronic sinusitis and eczema. I watched my ex-husband reverse his Lyme Disease. I've seen people age gracefully into their older years. The older people who are thriving in their health are the ones that inspire me the most. If you want to find health then you have to create healthy living habits. Seek out the healthiest people and see what they are doing. Question everything. Find mentors. The sooner you start the happier and healthier your life will be. We are designed to thrive in life. I believe in you. I want you to succeed on your health journey.

I have a deep love for people and I genuinely care about your well being. It has been hard for me to watch my parents health suffer. My mother has excellent health insurance and while I'm happy that she has this, I also think it gave her a false sense of security or a lack of accountability for her own health. She went to the best doctors and hospitals and spent millions of dollars on healthcare and I watch her suffer for years as she did this. I couldn't help but to think there had to be a better way. The one thing that she didn't try was to change her diet and lifestyle. She tried every surgery available to her and loads of prescription pills. She suffers from Crohn's Disease, Parkinson's, Edema and regular kidney stones. My dad has Alzheimer's and is already living in memory care at an assisted living home. His incontinence and wondering make it difficult to care for him at home with 2 children and work. Both my parents turn 70 this year and they are too young to be this sick. My father didn't change his diet or lifestyle either. I tried to be a positive influence on them. They say that nothing is learned unless the question is asked.

The beginning of my health journey began when I was pregnant with my daughter. I had a chronic sinus infection that lasted months and it was affecting my sleep. I chose to do a 10 day raw food detox at a Hypocrites Institute in Michigan. I did nothing but focus on eating healthy, learning about health and rest. I chose to do a detox verses take antibiotics to protect the health of my baby. Having children changed the course of my life. I wanted my children to live healthy lives. In my 20's health wasn't as important to me because I simply didn't know. When I was pregnant at 35 is when my life made a turn.

I grew up in a Standard American Diet home. We ate lots of meat and potatoes, almost every meal. When I was a kid I ate Campbell's Chicken noodle soup and a can of coke for breakfast everyday, Beef-O-Roni for lunch and meat and potatoes for dinner. We rarely ate vegetables that didn't come in a can and there was always a variety of processed foods. My mother grew up poor and wanted us to have the things that she couldn't have as a child. She had all the best intentions. She worked very hard to provide for us. I used to use decongestants on a regular basis and I used to get allergy shots one in each arm for five years. My allergies have significantly improved where I hardly notice them anymore. I lived on steroid cream as that was the only way I knew to relieve the itchy eczema that I had. I also got sick very often and constipated but not anymore.

Fruit was in our house when we grew up but during Chicago winters we weren't eating very much of it. I have four brothers so to make a dietary change in my life has been difficult as no-one in my family was eating the way I was. My health started to thrive and I'm glad that I made the changes that I did. I am able to concentrate much better because all the aches and pains no longer distracted me. It's amazing what we can accomplish when we feel good. My intention is to be a positive example so people are inspired to make healthy changes that can improve the quality of their lives. It is never too late to make a change and improve your health.

There is a law of limitations, however. For example, if I cut my arm, the cut will heal but it may leave a scar. My arm may never go back to the way it did before I injured it but it will heal to the best that the body can heal. The same healing happens on the inside of the body. The younger you are when you make a change the better as you can prevent a lot of damage from happening in the first place. Scar tissue happens on the inside of the body as it heals. The body will not injure itself and is always doing the best thing for itself. We need to trust that the body is this incredibly intelligent machine that is self-cleansing and self-healing. Take charge of your health as it will be one of the best investments that you ever make.

7 WALK AWAY FROM ANIMAL PRODUCTS AND DON'T LOOK BACK

Many people think we need animal protein for nutrition. This simply isn't true. We need amino acids and our bodies re-arrange these amino acids into usable proteins. Protein is used for growth and repair. As adults we are not growing much so it's mostly used for repair. An infant on a mono diet drinking nothing but breast milk will triple its size in one year. Human breast milk has less than 6 percent protein in it. That is the largest growth spurt of your life and you do it with less than 6 percent protein! As an adult you get all of the protein that you need from the whole foods that you eat. All whole foods have proteins, fats and carbohydrates, our three macro-nutrients, in the correct proportions that we need.

Another reason to avoid animal products is because they are acidic. A true carnivore's stomach has 7 times more hydrochloric acid than a human used to break down animal proteins, bones and organs. Humans have an alkaline digestive system including alkaline saliva and urine. We need an alkaline environment to thrive. Meat digestion requires our stomachs to increase the hydrochloric acidic in our stomach in order to properly break it down. This acid in our digestive track causes issues such as acid indigestion, upset stomach, constipation, heartburn and digestive disorders.

Disease thrives in an acidic environment. Even dairy is acidic. Not only that, dairy as a percentage of calories is a high fat food more than a high protein or high carbohydrate food. 2% Milk for example is 50% fat as a percentage of calories. The two percent is the weight of the fat in grams. If you convert those grams into calories and compare the same units of measurement then you will see that it is a 50% fat food. Cheeses are 70-80% fat. Eggs are high in cholesterol and fats. Eating fat foods are very enervating on the body forcing us to use nerve energy to break down fat into usable monosaccharides. Every cell in our body eats glucose remember. The proteins and fats contain complex molecules that take longer for your body to pull apart.

Meat has no fiber in it. Fiber is an essential nutrient, meaning that our bodies don't make it. Our bodies use fiber to absorb water from our bloodstream to help glide waste matter out of our bodies through peristalsis. Fiber is also used by our colons like a dumbbell. Our colons compress the fiber to keep the waste moving and exercising our colons properly amongst so many other benefits. Fiber goes in and out of our bodies so our bodies don't absorb it, we simply use it to move things on through while it helps to sweep our colons clean from any residue. Fiber is found in plants. It is the structure of the plant that holds it together. You can get all the fiber you need from eating plants. If you ever juice then you will see that the by-product is fiber. When we eat too much meat and dairy then it backs up in our system allowing toxins to get re-absorbed into the bloodstream when the toxic load is too large.

Humans have convoluted colons that are 12 times the length of our bodies verses a carnivore who has smooth colons that are only 3 times the length of their bodies. When we eat meat it takes a human much longer to digest animal proteins than a carnivore because we have less acid in our stomachs. Putrefactive byproducts can get stuck in a human convoluted colon and cause much havoc on our system. Literally we become full of shit. Ideally you want easy in, easy out foods. You don't want any waste products to linger.

Much of the meat we eat putrefies in our gut because it takes longer to move on through our bodies. Meat and fish can take as long as two days to fully digest. Imagine a steak sitting in a 98 degree oven for 48 hours. That's what happens inside your body. Putrefaction is the fifth stage of death used to break down proteins. Putrefaction breaks down the cohesiveness between tissues, and the liquefaction of most organs. The decomposition of organic matter happens by bacterial or fungal digestion, which causes the release of gases that infiltrate the body's tissues, and leads to the deterioration of the tissues and organs. Putrefaction inside the human body is not clean and the by-products are toxic.

Most meat doesn't even taste good without condiments on it such as salt, preservatives and sauces. All of these condiments are used to make plain food taste good. Our taste buds crave these condiments, not the meat.

Fruits and vegetables are high in fiber and move through your system in less than a day. These high-fiber foods help your digestive track run more efficiently. Bottom line, stay away from animal products for optimal health and never look back. Soon after it is gone, you won't even miss it. You will start to crave fresh fruits and vegetables especially as your pallet cleanses. Get the extra condiments out of your system, especially the salt. Salt deadens your taste buds and retains a lot of water weight. You will be able to taste your raw foods better once you give up salt and clean the pallet.

8 RAW OR COOKED?

The more raw foods that you eat the better. Cooked foods can be a secondary choice. I'm not saying don't eat them but I am saying that cooking destroys the nutrition in the food to varying degrees depending on the heat levels. The hotter the cooking, the more nutrition is destroyed. Lightly steamed vegetables and boiled sweet potatoes are not as harmful as deep frying foods. You ultimately get to decide at the end of the day. Just keep in mind that your body will respond to everything that you give it either positively or negatively. The information that I give you is simply for you to use as a tool so that you can make the best decisions for your health. My goal is to empower you.

Raw foods are the best for many reasons. Vitamins such as vitamin C are easily damaged by heat. Cooking cooks the water out of foods which forces you to drink more water to stay properly hydrated. Cooking cooks the flavor out of foods. Raw foods simply taste better. How often do you eat cooked food with nothing on it? Most importantly, your health will soar when you eat more raw fruits and vegetables. Make conscious choices about your health and you will be rewarded. I challenge everyone to try eating raw fruits, vegetables, nuts and seeds for 30 days and see how you feel. Now don't be surprised if you have detox symptoms if you do this but hang in there, natural healing takes time. You spent your whole life eating things that don't belong in your body so have some patience.

There are three main macro-nutrients in your body, carbohydrates, protein and fat. These three macro-nutrients are all impacted by cooking. Here are some examples. When you cook carbohydrates they caramelize. This is the brown color that you see on toast. That is a carcinogen or toxin in your body that is related to cancer. You also see this browning effect when you bake potatoes in the oven.

When you heat proteins then they get denatured. Imagine a piece of hair by a flame. The hair is high in protein and it curls and twists in ways that can't be put back together into its original form. Your body uses amino acids to build and restore the body not protein. When you eat protein, your body breaks down the amino acids and rearranges them in an order that your body can use. Now imagine two amino acids fused together because of heat. Your body doesn't know what to do with this fused amino acid and now it has to bring in white blood cells to remove them from your body. A high white blood cell count is used to clean infection. That's what you are doing with your body when you eat cooked protein, you are inflaming the body, literally. If you don't believe me then try this simple test for yourself. Eat very clean for a day and then get a blood test the following day. Now eat your Standard American Diet or better yet get a blood test the day after a big traditional Thanksgiving meal with lots of animal products and get a blood test and you will see your white blood cell count shoot up. Heavy meat eaters have puffy faces and bodies due to this inflammation. This enervates the body and it's not healthy.

Fats go rancid with heat. Rancid is the unpleasant smell or taste as a result of being old and stale. When you eat deep fried foods it is cooked in oil that is often not changed as much as you think. The reheating of oils makes the oil hydrogenate turning it into a transfat. This clogs up the arteries in the body making it more difficult to deliver oxygen to all the parts of the body that need it. Food companies put transfats into a lot of baked goods to stabilize the shelf life. Anything that is artificial, fake or used to increase a products shelf life is not food for you.

You don't want oxidation to happen on the outside of the body. An example is if you take a bite of an apple and that spot turns brown. That is oxidation. Food needs to oxidize inside the body. That's how our body breaks down the food and uses it as fuel. Now imagine eating a food that is preserved to not oxidize. That is a little weird for me. Mother Nature didn't mess it up. The laws of nature are simple, follow your instincts and you will be healthier.

9 EXERCISE - CONSISTENCY IS KEY

The best way to be consistent with your exercise is to find an activity that you enjoy. If you have joy and play when you exercise then it will be easy to sustain. I used to be in a professional dance company in my teens and I used to dance everyday at school instead of gym. I discovered yoga and I love trying new yoga postures. If I fall then I laugh at myself and try again. This simply means that I am learning something new and that I am growing. I don't take it too seriously but I am committed to it as I have been committed to some form of exercise for a large chunk of my adult life. I like that there is an endless amount to learn in yoga. You never actually get "there" because there is always more. This keeps my exercise interesting as there is always growth.

I can't stress the importance of consistency with exercise. Strength is built over time a little by a little. You don't have to work out for hours and hours everyday but I do recommend being smart and consistent with your workouts. If you are new to exercise then start slowly to prevent injuries and gradually increase the intensity of your workouts over time. I used to work out for over two hours a day before I made dietary changes but I was still a little chubby despite my hard work. I made the changes in my diet to a high raw, low fat whole food plant based diet and I saw that I had more energy for better workouts and faster recovery.

I used to run everyday and I was bad about stretching. Over time I developed severe plantar fasciitis. I would get sharp pain in my feet especially in the morning. I could barely walk, ouch! I switched to yoga, yin yoga and TRX and healed my plantar's feet. Yoga has progressions and can get very hard fast. I used to disregard it because I was a workout snob and I didn't think that I could burn as many calories as I could running. My yoga workouts are very intense and overall the number of calories from one sport to the other are comparable. For me I saw that I could have a longer sustaining athletic career as a yogi especially as I age verses a runner with better overall conditioning of my whole body. Now, if you are an avid runner, I'm not saying stop by any means. If you love it then keep doing it. Maybe you would like to add yoga into your routine to prevent injury and for muscle length. It really helped me tremendously. The thing that I like most about yoga is that it is exercise that is therapeutic for your body. It is designed to heal the body through yoga postures to stretch the fascia tissue in the body, to strengthen the muscles and to create healthy joints. I do yoga or TRX approximately 5 to 6 days a week.

Over the course of my exercise career I have done step aerobics, cardio-kick boxing, weights, cycling, running and calisthenics. I used to play volleyball, softball, snowboarding, golf, surfing and I was an avid dancer in my youth. I received an incredible benefit from all of these activities and I really love movement. It takes time to get in shape but it is not so hard to maintain it. The joy that I feel from being able to move my body pain free is wonderful and something that I hope to share with you all. I am 43 and I can move and push myself when I used to think that as you aged that your body somehow gives out on you. Age might slow you down but you will be surprised by what the body can do even in your older years.

I personally dedicate about 45-75 minutes a day exercising. Yes life gets busy and I will miss a day here and there but if I can get my exercise in then I will. I have made this commitment to myself. I feel very strongly that my daily exercise along with eating healthy is like putting money into my health bank. It is my natural anti-depressant and mood lifter. I like to ride my edge when I exercise so I can grow. I also don't push myself too far to avoid getting injured and if I do then I know to back off and slow down. The longevity of your exercise career is what matters most. If you don't exercise already then start. It is a critical component to your overall health and it will be one of the best investments you ever made. I wish you much joy and happiness as you move your body!

10 FASTING - MY EXPERIENCE WITH WATER ONLY FASTING

I have completed two water only fasts, one lasting 5 days and another lasting 14 days. I did both of these fasts unsupervised at home. The longer fast, I was communicating with my Natural Hygiene mentor on all of my symptoms for guidance. I am very happy that I took the time to water fast as a lot of healing took place.

During the 5 day water only fast I was still caring for my two children and lactating so I kept this fast to a shorter fast. The first 3 days of my 5 day fast I slept a big chunk of the day which makes me think that I could have been recovering from adrenal fatigue. I stopped having bowel movements after day 2. By day 4 I was feeling a lot better and I had a lot of energy. I exercised on day 1. I took a yoga class. I also did a light workout on Day 4. I did a 20 minute short run and a single set of light weights. I lost 8 pounds on this fast which was mostly water weight. I got my period during this fast and I was late. I am normally on a 28 day cycle and I got my period on day 34. Maybe the fast helped to straighten out my flow? Who knows. I did this fast because I wanted to eliminate a lot of bloating that I was receiving. The fast did help with this a lot. I became aware of how much I think about food. I was obsessed. I would often walk into the kitchen and open the refrigerator and close it. Fasting can bring up emotions from the past that we might not have thought of and many people including myself medicates our emotions with food.   It would be even better to sit with these emotions, process them and feel them so we can finally release them. Fasting helped me see this.

During the 14 day water only fast, I had intense detox symptoms that were challenging for me. Not eating for 14 days isn't so bad but the detox symptoms really tested my will.   My kid's daddy took the children to see their grandparents and I had 10 days alone. I really needed this downtime to recover.   I stopped having bowel movements after day 3. When I started the fast I weighed in at 134 lbs, after 5 days I dropped down to 126 lbs. At the end of the fast I dropped down to 116 lbs. I wasn't doing the fast for weight loss but for health. The weight loss is just something that will happen during a fast. After the fast, it is common to gain some of the weight back so don't be surprised. When I broke the fast it is important to eat clean and begin eating slowly. I had coconut water and 1/2 a papaya to break my fast.

I was really tired the first three days of the fast. Around day 5 I had intense back pain. The pain was shooting into my hips and the tops of my thighs. I couldn't even lie down because I was in so much pain. I had to sleep at a 90 degree vertical angle sitting upright. I suspect my kidneys were detoxing and causing this pain. When I was pregnant with my son, I developed varicose veins all down the back of my legs. After delivering the baby and losing weight, much of the veins went away.   I can't help but to believe that there were also toxins in my arteries preventing the blood to return from my lower extremities. This could have contributed to the pain in my low back, I'm not really sure. In the past I took a lot of pharmaceuticals as a child, I used to drink and I used to eat a Standard American Diet with lots of processed foods. I'm sure my kidneys were doing some major house cleaning.

I was teaching yoga classes but mostly calling out cues and demo'ing poses. Outside of this I really didn't exercise. I took this fast more seriously because I had the time off from being a mother and I wanted to maximize the benefits of healing my body. I didn't feel too hungry during the fast overall so that really didn't bother me. It just makes me see how we medicate ourselves with food. We think that we need to eat as much as we do but that's not really true. Many of our trips to the refrigerator are out of boredom or routine and not because we have a real feeling of hunger. Hunger is felt in the back of the throat and I didn't feel this the whole 14 day fast. When you don't eat, all of a sudden you have an incredible amount of time. A huge chunk of the day is spent, buying food, preparing food and cleaning up after food. I had so much less to do and was really able to focus. I was taking an online course on Natural Hygiene and was able to finish a few modules easily.

Around day 7 my sinuses kicked on for the rest of the fast and even two weeks after the fast. They were running non-stop with both of my nostrils completely blocked. Eventually the right nostril cleared. I had to have tissues by me all the time and I often had to sleep with my mouth open. Mucus is an export medium designed to export toxins out of the body so it makes sense that during a detox, my sinuses were draining a lot of mucus. Thankfully my sinuses lighten up near the end of my fast. Around day 8 I developed a lingering cough. I kept coughing up phlegm and I would spit it out so that these toxins got out of my body. I smoked in the past and I suspect that this was my body cleaning my lungs. My skin was really dry around my mouth and peeled off. This could have been from blowing my nose so much or new skin wanting to come through. My lips dried up and crusted over while feeling inflamed. If I smiled too big they would crack. Maybe this was from wearing lipstick or from smoking in the past? I didn't wear any makeup during the fast so who knows. My urine was super yellow while fasting.

At day 10, my kids, my 5 year old girl and my 3 year old boy and their daddy came home and the fast was more challenging for me because I had to make food for my kids and help take care of them. I couldn't rest as much as I would have liked during a fast and my son wanted to continue nursing. I was able to still nurse but my milk supply went down a lot and he was mostly nursing for comfort more than food at this point. The last four days of my fast, I was raising children and getting busier so I ended it. As a mommy, I'm simply grateful that I had the chance to fast. Mother's give so much for the family and it's easy to take care of ourselves last. We need to take time for ourselves so that we can better serve. We can't serve on an empty vessel. It is easier to fast when resting and not making food for others but we do the best we can.

The fast was a very spiritual time for me, especially since I was alone. I really cherish this alone time to rest, unwind, process and to listen. I had undistracted time to sit alone with my thoughts and witness what was going on in my head. I had a very emotional year with a divorce and this time allowed me to release some painful emotions. It's not uncommon to cry and release. When we hold these emotions in and don't allow ourselves to fully feel them then we are stuffing them down but they are still there. Many times we use our addictions to avoid dealing with our emotions, whether it be food, alcohol, drugs, sex, gambling or whatever we may use to comfort ourselves to avoid dealing with our feelings. None of this is healthy. Processing and feeling your feelings are necessary and healthy. It might hurt but eventually like all things they will pass and you will feel better and have a more grounded mind to avoid any addictive patterns. The whole point is to achieve a higher state of health and consciousness.

I became aware of unhealthy behavioral patterns that I have been repeating. Many of these patterns developed for survival due to various traumas throughout my life. Fasting gave me an awareness of this so I can end these patterns once and for all and come into a higher version of myself. It's painful to do shadow work and look at our own darkness but when we do this we are able to become friends with this dark side and use it as an ally in our lives instead of a place of fear that drives us into bad decisions. We are also given a chance to reconcile any relationships that have been hurt by these decisions through our conscious awareness of them. When we develop this awareness we can control our emotions and respond to things more thoughtfully and consciously instead of a knee jerk reaction to something that triggered us.

I noticed after my fast that I was able to perform at very high levels. Slowly but surely I was able to do more and more advanced yoga postures. My flexibility increased a lot. Maybe because whatever was going on in my low back has cleared up. My energy levels started to soar and I didn't have excess mucus to hold me back. My body was able to focus on my performance more than house cleaning. The benefits to the fast are amazing. Yes it is difficult but the results are worth it. Natural detox to health doesn't happen overnight. Whenever you eat poorly or healthy your body pays, either it suffers or benefits. You decide. A fast is the best way to do the fastest house cleaning on your body. You can go to a doctor supervised fasting center if you feel you need extra guidance or you can experiment on your own. The benefits of a fast compound over time the longer you are on a fast. Some people go as long as 25-40 days. I recommend having a mentor or some kind of supervision for a longer fast with someone with some experience.

I wish the road to health was easier but it's not and you do need some self-mastery and self discipline. Because of this, many people opt for the easy way out by taking medicine's. Unfortunately they will never get the results they are looking for taking this route. Health is caused by healthy living and a clean body. Medicines don't help to clean our bodies. Our bodies clean our bodies. All we need to do is get out of the way. Our bodies clean the most immediate concerns first and then goes on to work on the next most urgent issue. Our bodies are wicked smart and incredibly amazing. Your body is the most magnificent machine that you will ever know. The more that you learn about it and how to take care of it the better you will feel. Life is about joy, don't let an illness hold you back. Take the necessary steps to assist your body to reverse the damage that may have happened to it. Taking investment into your health is the best investment that you can make. We live in our bodies not in our fancy houses or fancy cars. Self care is the most unselfish thing that you can do. You deserve health, it is your birthright. You are capable of so much more than you can possibly imagine.

11 DEALING WITH ADDICTIONS

You may know the right things to do with your body but you may not be able to control your desires or urges therefore sabotaging your efforts. I think dealing with addictions is a huge humble step for everyone to move their health in a positive direction. I was in denial of my addictions to alcohol, marijuana and caffeine for a long time mostly because I didn't want to give them up. I loved these drugs, especially when I was feeling bad. The only problem was that these drugs did not love me back. I was able to eat better but it really took me a long time to deal with my addictions. I wanted to make the right choices but my mental and emotional body were wounded and they needed healing.

When I went through my yoga teacher trainings, I went through a mental, emotional and spiritual healing. As I did an incredible amount of self study on developing a higher consciousness, I found my addictions naturally falling away effortlessly. In the past it would take mammoth efforts for me to resist many urges that I somehow find easy now. I developed an incredible amount of self love and compassion through the power of forgiveness of others and especially myself. In yoga if we have a bad experience with something then it's called a samskara. A samskara is an impression on our mind that creates looping thought patterns. A samskara is usually a negative impression which we often cling to. When we deal with healing the mental and emotional body then we need to reveal these samskara's into our consciousness. When we become aware of them then we can awaken our consciousness, release the samskara and create better choices.

I was the queen of holding grudges, believe me but it didn't serve me at all. I lost time and people I love because I was concerned with being right. I was hurt and I wanted apologies. What I didn't also see was that I also was hurting people in the process of my righteousness. In my healing journey I said I was sorry to people that I love for my part of the relationship having any negative energy and that I love them. At the end of the day, I really do love them. Why was I so angry with them for so long? I needed to let things go. When I did it I found humble tears rolling down my face and an energetic weight lifted off of me. All of a sudden I felt lighter and happier. Everything changed for me. My whole life turned into a positive direction. I felt love for everyone especially myself.

Another thing that I learned was that "you are not special". Special compared to who? We are all the same. We all want love, family, friends and happiness in our life. One life is not more valuable than another life. This lesson served me as I started to observe the way people treated others. If I saw someone lying to one person then I knew that I'm not special and they would also lie to me. The same goes for ourself. If we are mean to others then we will also be mean to ourselves. Learn to find love for everyone and live your life with ethics. Be kind to people. Tell the truth. Live in the light. You will see everything in your life will become easier. Love will fill your heart and most importantly you will feel joy. Real joy that is unshakable. What is true will last.

Finally, find some kind of spiritual practice to whatever God that you believe in. Meditate. Set intentions. Pray. Find compassion. Ask for forgiveness and forgive others. What things have you done to hurt people and how have you tried to rectify them? You will find your whole world change yet it is the same. Energetically you will be traveling in joy verses pain and suffering. Your fears will fall away and you will see your worthiness. You all are so incredibly worth it. You all have infinite abilities to create endless amounts of beauty in this world. Heal yourself and do it!

12 PLANT BASED IS GOOD FOR OUR HEALTH, THE ANIMALS AND THE PLANET

I originally got into the plant based lifestyle because of health reasons. I saw so many friends and family dying, or suffering with illnesses.   I met people who were reversing their autoimmune diseases! This was amazing for me. I had my fair share of health issues to deal with and I wanted to feel better. I wanted this thriving health that I heard so many people claim. I was hungry for healing. Health is normal and natural. This is our natural state and our bodies will instinctively steer us into this direction. I wanted to heal my body and in the process I healed my mind. I mostly eat lots of fruits and vegetables and occasionally will eat cooked plant based foods. I have never felt better. My yoga practice has taken off and my energy levels are soaring.   As far as I'm concerned, changing my diet changed my life. I'm much happier now that I've ever been before. I went through a lot to make changes but if I can do it then so can you!

I saw how incredibly awful farm animals are treated. They are living beings that are trapped in small cages waiting to be turned into food. There's a reason why you never actually see how your food is made. It's because it is so god awful that most people wouldn't be able to stomach it. They are often abused, neglected, under exercised and malnourished. How many of you actually met a cow for example? They are gentle and kind the same as a dog. It baffles me how we can have such a high value for one animal and such a low value for another. Remember we are one. All animals feel pain, love their babies and have instincts for survival. They want to live and thrive the same as we do. I refused to watch those awful documentaries that showed the horror that the animals go through until one day I said I had to watch it to see how bad it was. I still see the faces of the animals being brutalized. It was way worse than anything I could imagine and I couldn't consciously eat meat after sitting through a film on the animals being tortured for our food. It's just not right. I challenge you to watch one of the documentaries about animal agriculture for yourself. Learn and become awake to what is going on.

80% of our monoculture grain crop goes to feed these farm animals. These monoculture crops are destroying habitats for wildlife. Think about an acre of land with nothing but corn growing on it. Now imagine spraying round up ready pesticides all over this corn. Round up ready pesticides kill everything in that acre except the patented round up ready corn seeds. This kills the ecology in an entire acre of land. Now imagine a fruit orchard. Imagine all the wild life that would thrive in this fruit orchard including the bugs, birds and micro-organisms. On top of that all, these pesticides get into our water supply. The way we are farming today is destroying our top soil and it is not getting replenished. The feces from the farm animals gets into our water supply creating algae blooms which suck all the oxygen out of the water creating dead zones. I can't think of anything worse than destroying our environment, while hurting animals that harm our health. They are all connected. It's time for our society to wake up and see that they have a choice at every grocery store visit to make a change in the world. If you care about animals, if you care about your health and your loved ones, if you care about global warming and the environment then wake up to the reality around you. You can make a difference!

13 GOODBYE BEAUTIFUL PEOPLE

I hope this book inspires you to live a healthier life. I want to share my passion for fruit with you all. I write a blog so if you would like to stay connected then you can check out my web page: selfhealinginspiration.com. selfhealinginspiration is my Instagram page and I also have a Self Healing Inspiration Facebook page. If you liked this book then please submit a positive review as it helps other people find this important message. Please send me a message if you have any comments on the book or my blog articles. Many blessings!

CONCLUSION

Thank you again for downloading this book! I have a lot of gratitude for each and every one of you.

I hope this book was able to help you to find Heath Through Fruit. I love hearing your stories, please share on my Facebook page for Self Healing Inspiration.

Finally, if you enjoyed this book, then I'd like to ask you for a favor, would you be kind enough to leave a review for this book on Amazon? It'd be greatly appreciated!

Thank you and good luck! Besos!

ABOUT THE AUTHOR

Amy Lynn Hager lives in Clermont, Florida with her two children and mother. Amy is originally from Chicago, Illinois where she has lived most of her life. She moved to Ecuador after her ex-husband got Lyme disease for six months and then moved to Clermont, Florida to be closer to her parents who lived in The Villages, Florida at the time. Her ex-husband and her split up but still maintain a positive and loving co-parenting relationship for their beautiful two children. Amy studied Finance at The University of Illinois Urbana/ Champaign. She found herself in a series of careers from 8 years in IT, broker/owner of Hendricks Realty, LLC, on-camera, theater & voice-over actress, dog trainer, 500 HR Certified Yogi and Mindset Coach. She has a Detox Certification with Dr Robert Morse, International School of Regenerative Detoxification. Never stop learning and keep exploring yourself. You never know what will grab at your heart in life until you live it fully.